# 12 METHODS OF BUILDING SEXUAL TENSION WITH A WOMAN.

## Basic seduction acts.

By

# Dr TIMOTHY KESSINGTON

approval from the publisher or creator.

# TABLE OF CONTENTS

ABOUT THE AUTHOR

INTRODUCTION.

# TABLE OF CONTENT

# ABOUT THE AUTHOR

**Dr. TIMOTHY KESSINGTON** is a licensed psychologist in the state of texas. he is a certified counselor on marriage and relationship/mental health. He is passionate to the core to see people in relationships happy and couples achieve the best out of every relationship

# INTRODUCTION

Building sexual tension is an important part of seduction, and it is a process that requires the right techniques and skills. You must learn how to create sexual tension if you want to attract a woman and keep her interested in you. This book  will teach you 12 different ways to create sexual tension with a woman.

# Chapter 1:

# Making Eye Contact.

Eye contact is an effective tool for increasing sexual tension. It is a nonverbal method of expressing your desire to a woman. Maintaining eye contact with a woman communicates that you are confident, assertive, and interested in her.

# CHAPTER 2

## Flirting.

Flirting is an important part of creating sexual tension. It entails playful and teasing communication that generates attraction and interest. Flirting can be verbal or nonverbal, and it is a subtle way to express your interest in a woman.

# CHAPTER 3

## Touch.


Touch is an important part of creating sexual tension. It can be an effective way to express your desire and attraction to a woman. Touch can be as simple as brushing up against her arm or hand or as intimate as a hug or kiss.

# Chapter: 4

## Body Language.

Body language is a nonverbal way of communicating to a woman your interest and desire. Posture, gestures, and facial expressions are examples of nonverbal communication. Using confident and assertive body language can help to create sexual tension and attraction.

# CHAPTER 5

## Verbal Communication.

Verbal communication is essential in creating sexual tension. It has to do with the words you use and how you say them. Using assertive and confident language can help to create a sense of attraction and sexual tension.

# CHAPTER 6

## Active Listening.

Active listening is an important part of creating sexual tension. It entails paying attention to what a woman says and responding in a way that demonstrates your interest in her. Active listening can aid in the formation of a connection and the creation of a sense of attraction.

# Chapter 7:

# Laughter.

Humor is an important tool for increasing sexual tension. It entails using humor to create an active and untroubled environment. Humor can help to relieve tension while also creating a sense of attraction and interest.

# CHAPTER 8

## The Unknown.

The element of mystery is a powerful tool for increasing sexual tension. It entails being unpredictable and leaving some things to the imagination. You can keep a woman interested and engaged by creating a sense of mystery.

# CHAPTER 9

## Flattery.

Flattery is a technique for increasing sexual tension by complimenting a woman. It entails finding compliments for her, such as her appearance, intelligence, or sense of humor. Flattery can elicit feelings of attraction and interest.

# CHAPTER 10

**Teasing**.

Teasing a woman is a playful way to increase sexual tension. It entails making fun of her in a lighthearted and playful manner. Teasing can arouse feelings of attraction and interest.

# CHAPTER 11

## Time Management.

When it comes to sexual tension, timing is everything. It entails knowing when to act and when to back down. You can create a sense of anticipation and sexual tension by being aware of the timing.

# CHAPTER 12

## Self-assurance.

Building sexual tension requires a high level of confidence. It requires you to be assertive and confident in your approach. You can create a sense of attraction and sexual tension by being confident.

# CONCLUSION

Building sexual tension is an important part of seduction, and it takes the right techniques and skills. Eye contact, flirting, touch, body language, verbal communication, active listening, humor, mystery, flattery, teasing, timing, and confidence are the 12 methods for increasing sexual tension with a woman.